Upgrade Your Temple

"The Faith and Fitness Guide to a Healthier and Happier You"

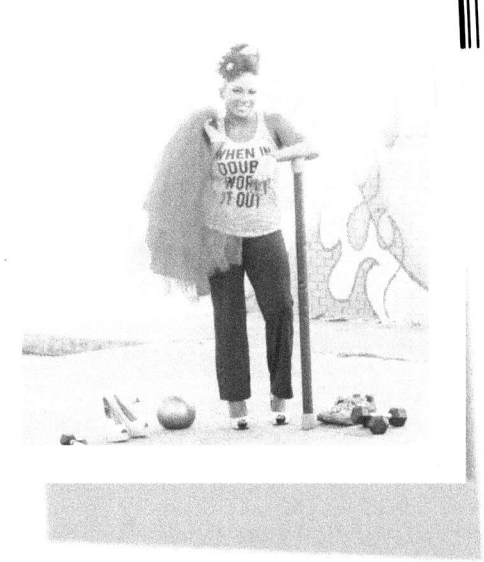

By: Dr. Kendra Mayes

Upgrade your Temple: Table of Contents

Kingdom Fitness Motto: "A fit Life is a Long Life"

Introduction

As, a fitness professional, I've noticed that planning, consistency and dedication to a fitness program seems to be increasingly difficult for people. They find themselves on the hamster wheel, going in circles as fast as they can, for a short amount of time, but making little to **NO** progress. Through this guide I want to encourage you to remain committed and dedicated to the personal cause of healthier living. Keep doing what it takes to accomplish your goals along with incorporating health, wellness, and spiritual wholeness into all that you do, on a daily basis.

Philippians 4:13: "I can do all things [which He has called me to do] through Him who strengthens *and* empowers me [to fulfill His purpose—I am self-sufficient in Christ's sufficiency; I am ready for anything and equal to anything through Him who infuses me with inner strength and confident peace.]

Living in such a fast pace society can be a challenge; the added pressure stemming from responsibilities personally and professionally can cause frustration with maintaining a lifestyle change. The heaviness of trying to successfully manage a work/life balance can become a fading thought. Often questions merge like how will I get started? When will I ever have time? Will I have enough money to sustain the change? Who can I depend on to support this new change in my life? These questions and life's challenges are real.

Don't beat yourself up! Instead it's important to remember that you are important! You are worthy of having a long life! Just as you didn't gain weight or become unhealthy overnight, you are not going to lose weight or establish healthier lifestyles overnight. This journey is a process that requires patience and perseverance physically, mentally, and spiritually. Research suggests it takes anywhere from 21-40 days to build new habits. Learning new habits, establishing balance, and reconnecting with your health and wellness goals are all possible.

The journey to a healthier and happier life is not about perfection, but progress. If you want a happier, healthier, and fulfilling life the change must begin with you. This book will provide practical tips to help ignite your journey to a healthier and happier you. This book will also serve as a book of reflection allowing you to journal your thoughts, so in those times of discouragement you can read over your amazing accomplishments.

What's On Your Plate?

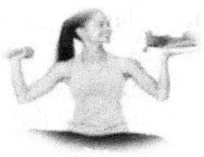

A balanced diet is essential in leading a healthy lifestyle, and can help or hinder your health and wellness journey. It's important to examine your food habits, what foods give you energy and what foods make you feel sluggish, sleepy or tired. The proper fuel is important to the body. The proper fuel determines how well we function throughout the day. When the body is not fueled properly you increase your chances of fatigue, poor performance, and disproportionate weight size. Additionally, being conscience about your nutritional intake, is equally as important in not only managing weight but also in the reduction of common diseases such as diabetes, hypertension, cholesterol, heart disease and even cancer.

When leading a busy life style, monitoring your food intake will be a pillar to your success. If you feel like you are running low on energy or seem unable to complete what you've started.

Consider making the following changes to your diet:

> ➤ Minimize processed foods and surgery snacks, replace with fruits, veggies, whole grain snacks, and water.
> ➤ Incorporate meatless days. This is a great way for the body to detox, incorporate protein by adding beans, lean meats, eggs, and turkey, or soy to your diet.
> ➤ Consider adding in a "green day", to fill the body with vegetables such as kale, spinach and cucumbers, to boost your metabolism, and mood.

Daily Affirmation: "If you don't go within, you go without!"

Diet Meditation

1 Corinthians 6:12: All things are lawful for me," but not all things are helpful. "All things are lawful for me," but I will not be enslaved by anything.

1. How do you think your current food intake affects your daily performance?

   _____

   _____

   _____

   _____

2. How often in a week do you have fast food?

   _____

   _____

   _____

   _____

3. What could you do differently for the upcoming week?

   _____

   _____

   _____

   _____

Did You Plan and Prepare?

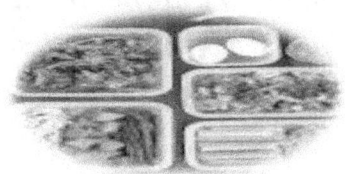

Meal prep is a great tool to stay organized and on track with your health and wellness goals. When leading a busy life it's important to keep the proper snacks readily available to prevent the vending machine raid. Take time to invest in prepping for the week. The benefit of preparing your meals and snacks allows you to save a considerable amount of calories, time, and money.

Once you make this a weekly habit, you won't be able to live without it. And the best part is you decide what works for you. The key is carving out time to prep your meals and maintain the process.

Here are some ideas to help you get started:

> ➢ If breakfast and lunch are a struggle, consider, focusing on prepping 2 days of meals. Multitask, while making your nightly dinner by preparing your breakfast and lunch for the next day or two until you develop a full routine.
> ➢ Cook stretchy meals so that you can freeze the leftovers for a later serving.
> ➢ Purchase on the go portion controlled snacks such as nuts, yogurt, and hard boiled eggs. These snacks are easy to prep, pack, and consume while leading a busy life.
> ➢ Get in the habit of washing and bagging fresh fruits and vegetables, so that they are easily assessable when needed.

Daily Affirmation: I will allow God to organize my time today, so that I may accomplish His will today!

Meal Planning and Preparation Meditation

Hebrews 12:11: For the moment all discipline seems painful rather than pleasant, but later it yields the peaceful fruit of righteousness to those who have been trained by it.

1. During the week what do you consider to be time wasters? How can you incorporate meal planning into those spaces?

_____

_____

_____

_____

2. How many times did you take leftovers for lunch?

_____

_____

_____

_____

3. What could you do differently for the upcoming week to better prepare for your health and wellness journey?

_____

_____

_____

_____

Eating Less is "MORE"

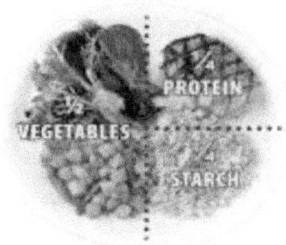

Eating on the go can be quite a challenge for maintaining a healthy lifestyle. Typically, restaurants offer larger portions of food and it seems as if every drive through attendee ask you to up size, super-size, or add a calorie dripping dessert. However, developing the habit of eating 5-6 smaller meals which consist of 3 meals and 2-3 smaller snacks a day is a great way to start concentrating on portion control. When you feed the body more frequently, the desire to over eat minimizes.

Here are some tips to help you get started with controlling those portions:

> Ask for a togo container when your restaurant entrée arrives. Splitting the entrée in half will, save you calories and reduce the temptation of over eating. Not to mention, 1 meal has just become 2 meals which helps you to save money!
> Skip the appetizer. Most of the time we don't realize how many calories we've consumed by ordering an appetizer, main entrée, and desert. Limit your options by choosing the most important food entrée.
> Eat on an 8-10inch plate at home verses a 12 inch plate. When eating on a larger plate you are actually doubling the normal serving size.
> Balance your meal consumptions. For example, if you have a larger breakfast than consider reducing your lunch and dinner portions.
> Drink a glass water 30 mins before each meal which helps to curb the appetite, enabling you to feel full before eating.

Daily Affirmation: My appetite will not control me, I submit all unhealthy and unwanted cravings

to God.

Eating Less is "MORE" Meditation

1 Corinthians 10:31: So, whether you eat or drink, or whatever you do, do it all to the glory of God.

1. Count how many times you've eaten today. Record what you've consumed? Where the meals healthy?
    a. Meal One:
    b. Meal Two:
    c. Meal Three:
    d. Meal Four:
    e. Meal Five:

    _____
    _____
    _____
    _____

2. How late was your dinner?

    _____
    _____
    _____
    _____

3. What could you do differently for the upcoming week to plan your healthy meals and design your eating schedule?

    _____
    _____
    _____
    _____

Exercise is the Spice of Life

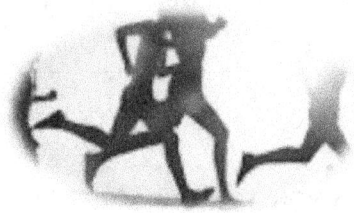

Doctors recommend the average person workout a minimum of 3-5 times a week for 30 minutes. I want to challenge you to look for an opportunity to work out! Working out has been linked to increasing self-image, academic performance, and mental stability. Working out also has been known to decrease depression, anxiety, obesity, cancer, diabetes and other health related illnesses that are prevalent in our current society. Exercise is a great way to decrease stress levels. Additionally, physical fitness has been associated with releasing feelings of happiness.

Take the practical approach to designing your workout regime (or consider implementing a regimen). For example, write down specific days that you would like to work out and divide your workout into 15 minute increments.

A few tips include utilizing:

- Make an appointment with yourself
- Maximize Commercial breaks
- At work take the stairs instead of the elevators
- Park far away when you are running errands.
- You can use your home, street, stairs, garage, or family room as a workout space. Where there is space there is opportunity

Daily Affirmation: "My body is a temple of God, so I am determined to increase my endurance, strength, and help through fitness. Today, I will pick my level and train with a spirit of excellence".

Determine to Exercise Meditation

1 Corinthians 9:27: I discipline my body like an athlete, training it to do what it should. Otherwise

1. How do you think exercising benefits you?

   _____

   _____

   _____

   _____

2. What are some things that prevent you from exercising?

   _____

   _____

   _____

   _____

3. What could you do differently for the upcoming week to better plan and prepare to implement 3 consistent days of 30 minutes of physical fitness into your week?

   _____

   _____

   _____

   _____

Explore the Out Doors

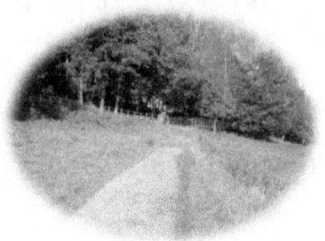

Always keep your workout shoes with you! The outdoors is a canvas that is often underused. Sometimes with the hustle of life, we simply forget to stop and smell the roses. You are encouraged to maximize your health and wellness journey by fully occupying all spaces that are provided.

For example, go for walks on your breaks or complete a quick lunchtime fitness circuit. Physical activates have been known to improve your mood, focus, and provide a nice boost of energy for the day. Some of the benefits of outdoor exercises include:

Benefits of the Outdoors:

> - Easily accessible for a quick stress reliever
> - Cost effective if you cannot afford a gym membership
> - It allows you the freedom to be you! No judgment zone.
> - The sun provides natural vitamin D which is good for the bones and skin
> - The entire family can join in.

Daily Affirmation: Today is the day that I will bask in the rays of the SON. I will enjoy the fresh air, the beautiful landscape, the birds singing, and the sounds of nature.

Motivated to Move Meditation

Isaiah 40:29: He gives power to the faint, and to him who has no might he increases strength.

1. How often do you exercise outside?

    _____

    _____

    _____

    _____

2. What are some simple activities that you could do outside?

    _____

    _____

    _____

    _____

3. What could you do differently for the upcoming week to make better use of the outdoors?

    _____

    _____

    _____

    _____

Support Sustains

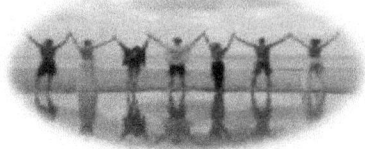

Social media, computer technology, and the community can offer you a variety of health and wellness support. All you have to do is plug in! Fitness is a great way to build positive relationships. Connect with online fitness teams or link up with your friends using fitness pal as a source of motivation and accountability.

Make fitness apart of your family by regularly visiting the local parks, take the dog for a walk, play outside with your children, or go for a bicycle ride or hike. The more you become involved with other people the greater the support, motivation, and ultimate results.

Benefits of Support Teams:

> ➢ Helps you to overcome weightless plateaus
> ➢ Keeps fitness fun and interesting
> ➢ Provides a source of healthy competition and challenge
> ➢ Increasing mental strength
> ➢ Greater source of encouragement

Daily Affirmation: I will committee myself to helping others maintain their health and wellness journey.

Support Sustains Meditation

Ecclesiastes 4:9: Two are better than one, because they have a good return for their labor: If either of them falls down, one can help the other up.

1. Are you currently connected to any fitness support groups? If not why?

_____

_____

_____

_____

2. How do you think a health and wellness support team would benefit you?

_____

_____

_____

_____

3. Who do you know that is serious about their health and wellness journey? Are you willing to take the lead and encourage others to get fit?

_____

_____

_____

_____

Attitude Adjustment

Your attitude toward leading a healthy life style can definitely impact your results. If you view your lifestyle change as a burden, then you will sabotage your own journey. There is no burden to be perfect on this journey. This is a lifelong process with the goal of being healthy and whole. Start now practicing gratitude and replace the "I cant's" with the "I can". Purchase a fitness journal so that you can write and reflect over your thoughts.

Celebrate both scale and non-scale victories. Change your thoughts, change your results, you are an investment. Creating a positive affirmation cycle for yourself will serve as a reminder that you are worth it. Becoming active and fueling your body with the proper nutrition, you are increasing your quality of life by adding more life to your days.

Benefits of Journaling:

- ➤ Great time of reflection
- ➤ Shows your progress
- ➤ Allows you to freely note your feelings
- ➤ Healthy way to increase yourself esteem and confidence

Daily Affirmation: I am fearfully and wonderfully made by God. I am working diligently to strengthen my temple so that I may be of greater value to the Kingdom of God. I will continue to THINK, SPEAK, AND ACT POSTIVE about my health and wellness journey. And each day I am making progress. I can and I will succeed.

Keeping a Positive Attitude
Meditation

Proverbs 23:7: For as he thinketh in his heart, so is he.

1. How do you think your attitude towards maintaining a healthy lifestyle impacts your results?

_____

_____

_____

_____

2. What are some ways you could improve your attitude?

_____

_____

_____

_____

3. What could you do differently for the upcoming week to have a better attitude towards your health and wellness journey?

_____

_____

_____

_____

Water Does a Body Good

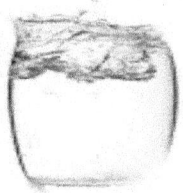

Water makes up 55 -65% of the body, which means water, is an essential part of our health and wellness journey! Water provides the body with excellent benefits. Increasing your water intake not only improves your brain function by minimizing confusion but also by flushing toxins, fat, and impurities from your system.

Water is a natural energy booster and is great for the skin and heart. Staying hydrated also aids in minimizing unwanted cravings. Water speeds up the metabolism and contributes to the overall health wellness and weight loss journey. Research recommends that individuals need to consume at least 6-8 glasses of water daily. DRINK YOUR WATER!

Benefits of Drinking Water:

- ➢ Increases oxygen within the body
- ➢ Flushes fat and toxins
- ➢ Replenishes skin
- ➢ Regulates PH balance
- ➢ Curbs appetite

Daily Affirmation: Today, I will make water a priority. I purify my body of all toxins by drinking the adequate amount of water.

Drink More Water Meditation

Daniel 1:11-13&15: Daniel then said to the guard whom the chief official had appointed over Daniel, Hananiah, Mishael, and Azariah, 'Please test your servants for ten days: Give us nothing but vegetables to eat and water to drink. Then compare our appearance with that of the young men who eat the royal food and treat your servants in accordance with what you see'. At the end of the ten days, they looked healthier and better nourished than any of the young men who ate the royal food."

1. How much water do you drink daily?

   _____

   _____

   _____

   _____

2. What prevents you from drinking the recommend amounts of water daily?

   _____

   _____

   _____

   _____

3. Find different detox water recipes to keep water interesting and a part of your wellness journey?

   _____

   _____

   _____

   _____

Rest is "Good" for the Soul

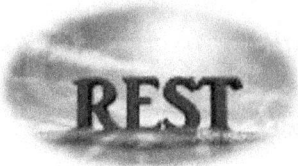

The recommended amount of sleep is 6-8 hours. The body needs time to recuperate and recover from the day's activities. Resting allows your mind and body to replenish and recover for the next day. Getting the adequate amount of rest also has positive health benefits.

The body normally burns between 100-200 additional calories in a rested state. Implementing a nightly bed time helps to prevent unwanted cravings. Often you are tempted to engage in unhealthy snacking when you are in a state of fatigue, thus consuming unnecessary calories, ultimately leading to weight gain.

Benefits of Resting:

➢ Refreshes the body
➢ Reduces fatigue
➢ Increases memory
➢ Curbs appetite

Daily Affirmation: A healthy body is a rested body!

Rest is "Good" for the Soul
Meditation

Psalms 4:8 In peace I will lie down and sleep, for you alone, LORD, make me dwell in safety.

1. How many hours of sleep do you average?

    _____

    _____

    _____

    _____

2. What prevents you from getting the adequate amount of sleep at night?

    _____

    _____

    _____

    _____

3. What could you do differently for the upcoming week to have a better week of rest to remain happy and healthy?

    _____

    _____

    _____

    _____

Live, Love, and Laugh

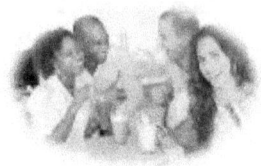

Living, loving, and laughing are essential to keeping your emotions and stress levels in check. Relaxation is a great way to escape from the demands of life. Apart of regaining your health and wellness, is taking time to live, love, and laugh. Laughter has been known to lower such conditions as stress and heart disease.

Make it a regular practice to decompress by scheduling in time to see a funny movie, quality time with family without working, take a weekend trip, or simply lounge around at home. The main focus is to become whole mind, body, soul, and spirit!

Benefits of Relaxing:

- ❖ Increase happy endorphins
- ❖ Maintains healthy and positive relationships
- ❖ Reduces tension, anxiety and stress
- ❖ Allows the body time to recuperate from vigorous activities relating to exercise

Daily Affirmation: The joy of the Lord is my strength, I will live, love and Laugh!

Relaxation Meditation

Genesis 2:2 And on the seventh day God came to the end of all his work; and on the seventh day he took his rest from all the work which he had done. How many hours of sleep do you normally average?

1. When is the last time you watched a movie with your family and or friends?

_____

_____

_____

_____

2. How often do you attend social events with family and friends?

_____

_____

_____

_____

3. What could you do differently for the upcoming week to incorporate a day of love and laughter with family and friends?

_____

_____

_____

_____

Mental Toughness

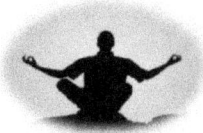

In a life that is filled with demands and expectations, taking time to cleanse our thoughts is important. Our thoughts have a way of controlling our actions. If we are frustrated, fatigued, angry, sad, mad, overwhelmed or confused then typically we are not motivated to carry out our daily task. It is in those very moments where you need to take a moment to meditate. Meditation has no right or wrong format. The purpose is to center your thoughts and energy into a state of calmness. Mediation should be a part of your daily routine. It's important to find time to collect yourself. Meditation can serve as a quick jump start to your mental and physical battery, which makes you stronger and emotionally sound. Meditation can be done to soft music or thinking about thoughts that make you happy.

Meditation can be as simple as a quick 2-3 minute stretch accompanied by deep breathing exercises. You can carve out 5-10 minutes of quite time on your breaks to just escape from the world. Meditation is a practice that can be done in simple spaces such as your home, car, outside, or where you designate as an adequate space.

Benefits of Mediation:

- Lowers blood pressure
- Increases energy levels
- Reduces anxiety
- Releases happy endorphins
- Helps you to gain clarity
- Provides peace of mind
- Enhances mental stability and sharpness
- Helps you regain focus

Daily Affirmation: Today, I will strengthen my mind, heart, and spirit by meditating on the word of God

Mental Toughness Meditation

Philippians 4:8 Finally, brothers and sisters, whatever is true, whatever is noble, whatever is right, whatever is pure, whatever is lovely, whatever is admirable—if anything is excellent or praiseworthy—think about such things.

1. How much time do you spend in a quiet place reading the word and listening to Gods Voice?

   _____

   _____

   _____

   _____

2. How do you think 15-30 minutes of meditation a day would benefit you?

   _____

   _____

   _____

   _____

3. What could you do differently for the upcoming week to designate a consistent time for meditation?

   _____

   _____

   _____

   _____

Making a Difference

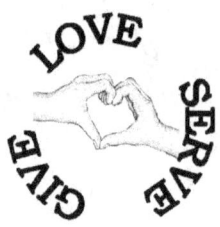

We make a living by what we get. We make a life by what we give. ~Winston Churchill~

Seeding and sowing should always be a part of your life. Those who make it a priority to be selfless are never without. It's been proven through countless research articles that those who spend money on others rather than themselves are happier. Acts 20:35 reminds us that it's better to give than to receive. Meaning we should always seek opportunity to make a difference in the lives of others. We are living in a world filled with giving opportunities. The selfless act of giving is God's way of showing care and compassion for those who need help, who are lost, and who need guidance.

As we look at poverty, literacy, displacement, and identity crisis the harvest is plentiful. It's time to take your eyes off of yourself and your issues and GIVE! Give time in mentoring, give time in charity, give in resources, and give a kind word. Find a way to show love, care and compassion to others. Giving has a way of making a powerful difference between life and death in the spirit, for not only the receiver but for you the giver. Research suggests that the power of giving a simple huge can be life changing! I challenge you to make a difference; you will feel better and be happier.

Benefits of Giving:

> ➢ Self fulfillment
> ➢ Happiness
> ➢ Personal Growth and enrichment

Daily Affirmation: God has called me to be part of something greater than myself. So, today, I am determined to make a difference on purpose.

Determined to Made a Difference Meditation

Luke 6:38 Give, and it will be given to you. A good measure, pressed down, shaken together and running over, will be poured into your lap. For with the measure you use, it will be measured to you.

1. Are you apart of any local chartable programs? How often do you volunteer or donate to a "cause" greater than you?

   _____

   _____

   _____

   _____

2. How do you think volunteering in faith based or community activities would enrich your life?

   _____

   _____

   _____

   _____

3. What could you do differently for the upcoming week to increase your level of giving (time, talent, professional service, finances)?

   _____

   _____

   _____

   _____

Points to Ponder

Your health and wellness spiritual journey is a lifelong commitment with no expiration date! You must remain on high alert and vigilant about the things that you consume. Ask GOD to quicken your spirit to the fatty, unhealthy, and salty foods, relationships, conversations, and activities that are in your life! And start feasting on the word of GOD more to help you overcome those cravings!

1. In order for you to shed the weight you need to check your diet. Fitness professionals suggest that when you seek to lose weight it is 70 percent diet and 30 percent exercises. It doesn't matter how much you workout if you are not consuming the right foods you only experience minimum results. When examining your food consumption you are advised to stay away from fast foods, fried food, and salty foods. Please understand that junk in…leads to junk out! You are encouraged to increase your proteins, fruits, vegetables and water which will lead you to greater results.

2. You must exercise in conjunction to changing your diet. Exercise is known to have physical, emotional, and spiritual benefits. Exercise causes our blood vessels to expand which is good for the heart, it challenges the body by producing sweat while getting rid of unhealthy toxins, and it helps to maintain weight control, improve our moods, and decrease unhealthy conditions. It provides an extra boost of energy and improves our sleep.

3. Support is also a great component in helping to get fit and taking out the trash in your life! When you join any fitness program one of the number one questions is who is your support team? This question is important because your environment is critical to your success. Support groups are known to help you to deal with your emotions, learning how to relieve stress, depression and anxiety. Support groups provide advice and feedback, along with being a network connecting to other people with the same goals and ambition. Support groups help you understand that you are not alone. The right kind of support group gives you life coaching and accountability.

4. Create purpose in your life by trimming the fatty areas of your life. God is with you and we are reminded in the word of God that we can do all things through his strength! It's time to sore to new heights, accomplish new goals, and live a better life. Make it your purpose to get rid of those things that are holding you down. You are encouraged to increase not only your physical exercise but your kingdom work. Set your goals and aim high. Take the time to meditate and love on yourself. And watch the pounds begin to shed physically, spiritually, and emotionally!

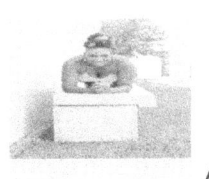

A Note From Dr. K

I am Dr. Kendra Mayes and I am a native of Fort Worth Texas. I am a personal trainer and the CEO of Kingdom Fitness, INC located in Fort Worth Texas. Our motto is" *A Fit Life is a Long Life*", I am also a community partner serving as a motivational speaker and faith and fitness conference facilitator. I work with multiple fitness facilities throughout the Metroplex as a Fitness instructor and Personal trainer.

I will advise any person seeking to lose weight to find a program that they not only like but also has a built in support system. Having support forges accountability, new friendships, and fitness camaraderie which are invaluable. Starting and maintaining a health and wellness journey is not a race it's a journey which doesn't require perfection but progress.

For this reason, I have championed the cause of health and wellness in the African American community. I serve as a spokes person, blogger, and advocate for weight loss. I was featured in the June 2015 issue **of Black Women Lose weight** which is an online weight loss magazine. I recently published an article entitled **"A Fit life is a long life: Consistency is Key"** in Nia Magazine (www.niamagazine.com) which is an online lifestyle and empowerment magazine for today's Black woman. I share with people practical principals of losing weight, selecting a fitness regimen, and maintaining their goals. On your new journey, give time, time! Maintain consistency; make a date with your gym or fitness group. And have fun trying new foods, new workouts, and making new friends!

Resources:	Kingdom Konnect:
www.google.com\images	Facebook: KingdomfitnessbydrK
www.crosswalk.com	IG Handle: KINGDOMFITNESS_DRK
International sports sciences association	http://kingdomfitness-dr.com

Beginners Lifestyle Change Plan

Starting a healthier lifestyle requires organization and planning with purpose!

Note: Before starting any lifestyle change programs please consult with your physician. This page is meant only to guide you on how to get started with your health and wellness journey.

Example workout schedule:

Monday Glutes	Tuesday	Wednesday Abs	Thursday	Friday Arms
10 squats 10 lunches (each leg) 10 back leg lifts (each leg) 10 fire hydrants (each leg) 10 donkey kicks (each leg)	30 min: Walk Run Cardio Dance	20 crunches 20 sit-ups 20 front leg extensions 1 min plank 1 min mountain climbers	30 min: Walk Run Cardio Dance	30 arm circles 10 push-ups 20 dip kicks 20 triceps kickbacks 1 min punches

Note: As your endurance increases change your routines and increase your workout times.

Example balance nutrition ideas:

Proteins	Carbohydrates	Vegetables	Fruit/Snacks
Chicken (Grilled or baked) **Tuna** **Fish (blackened, grilled, baked, pan sautéed)** **Lean Beef** **Turkey** **Beans** **Eggs**	Wheat pasta Brown rice Red, purple, white, or sweet potatoes	Kale Spinach Green beans Okra Broccoli Zucchini Squash Cauliflower Greens	Greek yogurt Peanuts Bananas Oranges Berries Apples Pineapples

Note: It's a good idea to play with a variety of foods and spices to see what you like. If you are in the weight loss phase these food are recommend as a basic way to get you started with changing your eating habits.

Example Meal Schedule:

7:00am	Breakfast
9:00am	Snack 1
12:00pm	Lunch
2:00pm/3:00pm	Snack 2
6:00pm/7:00pm	Dinner

Note: Consuming 5 meals a day prevents the body from going into starvation mode. Additionally by consuming food regularly your increasing the body's metabolism, meaning it burns nutrition higher and releases toxic waste quicker. You can adjust your 2-3 hour window for food during the day based on your schedule. However you are encouraged to have your last meal by 7pm which allows the body enough time to digest the meal properly.

Hydrate Feel great:

As discussed previously water is essential to your health and wellness journey. You should try with every effort to drink at least 1 gallon of water daily. This will help you fight cravings while flushing fat! Water does not have to be boring. Below are some basic fat flush water recipes. Also, feel free to research more and add variety even to your water!

1. Lemons, Limes, Oranges,-tap water
2. Lemons and Limes-tap water
3. Lemons, Limes, Cucumbers, Raspberries, Grapefruit, 2 mint leaves-tap water
4. Lemons, Limes, Raspberries- tap water
5. Lemons, Limes, Oranges, Grapefruit-tap water
6. Lemons and Apple Cider Vinegar- tap water

****Pack your water with all the ingredients*** Squeeze some of the fruit in the water for initial flavor then just add the rest…will automatically flavor the water****

****32oz fat flush on the go is good for about 3 days and multi refills**** the larger home refrigerated version (pitcher) is good for about a week….the older the better! The water will change color from all of the ingredients.*****

Meditation time is important:

Target at least 7 mins a day to meditate on God's word to refresh, refill, and renew your thoughts! Meditation will help to keep you motivated about being healthy and fit. Consider these additional scriptures to aid you in your meditation time:

1. "May the very God of peace sanctify you completely. And I pray to God that your whole spirit, soul, and body be preserved blameless unto the coming of our Lord Jesus Christ" (1 Thess. 5:23).

2. "I can do all things because of Christ who strengthens me" (Phil 4:13).

3. "So, therefore, I run, not with uncertainty. So I fight, not as one who beats the air. But I bring and keep my body under subjection, lest when preaching to others I myself should be disqualified" (1 Cor. 9:26-27).

4. "Therefore, whether you eat, or drink, or whatever you do, do it all to the glory of God" (1 Cor. 10:31).

5. "What? Do you not know that your body is the temple of the Holy Spirit, who is in you, whom you have received from God, and that you are not your own?" (1 Cor. 6:19).

6. "but those who wait upon the Lord shall renew their strength; they shall mount up with wings as eagles, they shall run and not be weary, and they shall walk and not faint" (Is. 40:31).

7. "She clothes herself with strength, and strengthens her arms" (Prov. 31:17).

8. "Now no discipline seems to be joyful at the time, but grievous. Yet afterward it yields the peaceful fruit of righteousness in those who have been trained by it. Therefore lift up your tired hands, and strengthen your weak knees" (Heb. 12:11-12).

9. "You are of God, little children, and have overcome them, because He who is in you is greater than he who is in the world" (1 John 4:4).

10. "No temptation has taken you except what is common to man. God is faithful, and He will not permit you to be tempted above what you can endure, but will with the temptation also make a way to escape, that you may be able to bear it" (1 Cor. 10:13).

11. "Thus I do not run aimlessly; I do not fight as if I were shadowboxing. No, I drive my body and train it, for fear that, after having preached to others, I myself should be disqualified." (1 Cor 9:26-27)

12. "He gives power to the faint, abundant strength to the weak. Though young men faint and grow weary, and youths stagger and fall, they that hope in the LORD will renew their strength, they will soar on eagles' wings; They will run and not grow weary, walk and not grow faint." (Isaiah 40:29-31)

13. "I have competed well; I have finished the race; I have kept the faith." (2 Timothy 4:7)

The Journey

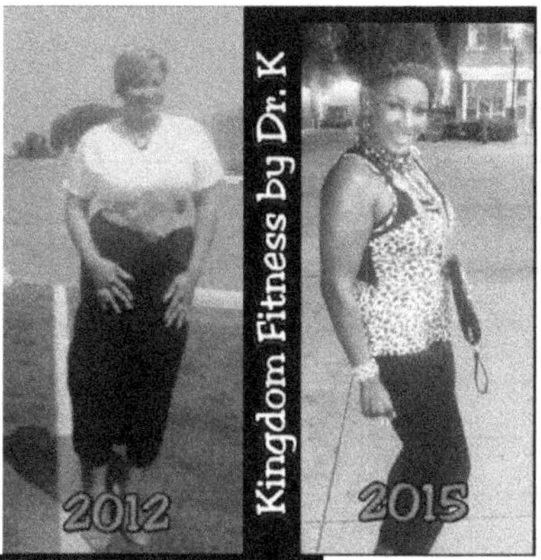

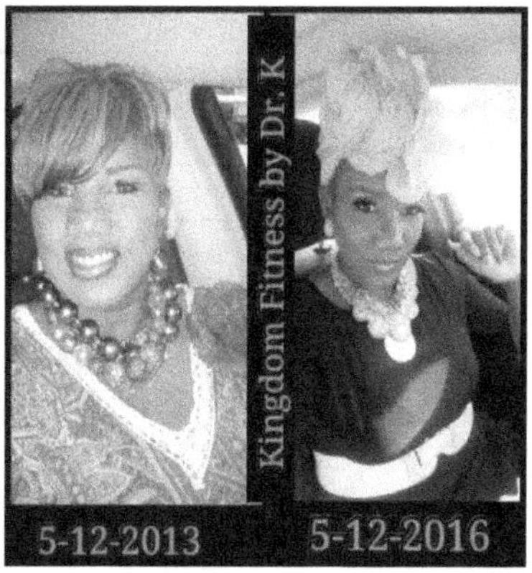

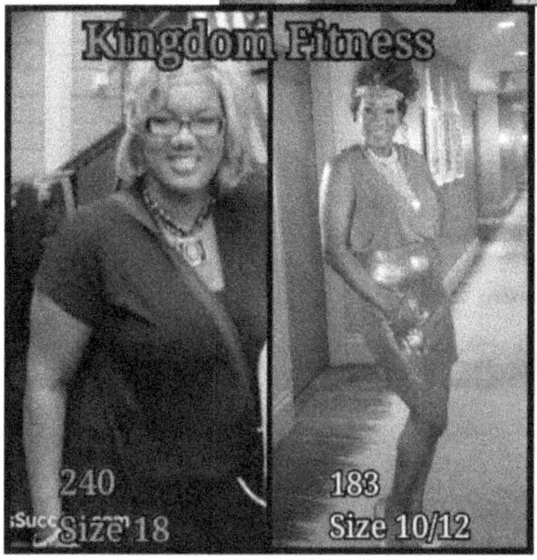

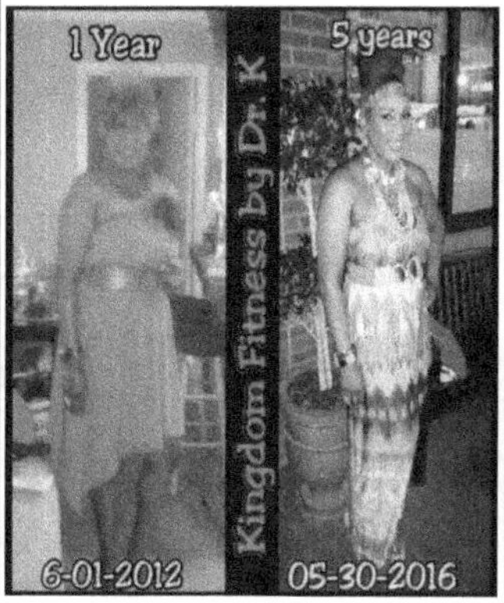

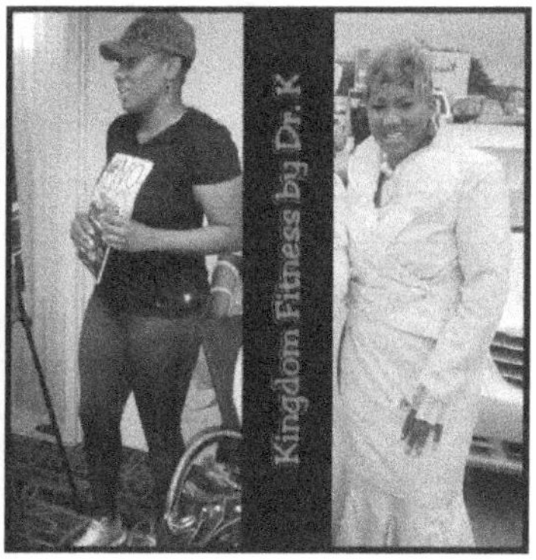

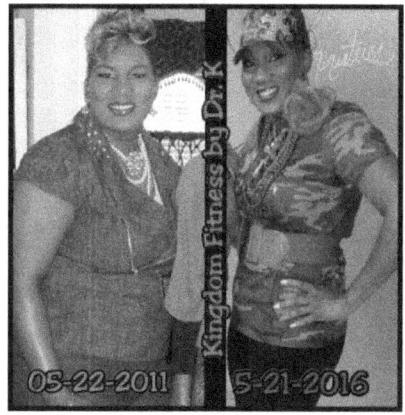

Kingdom Fitness Motto: "A fit Life is a Long Life"

Journal Your Thoughts